THE STUBBORN FAT CURE

By

Danial Barron Howe

Get The Book That Started a Revolution!

http://bit.do/the30dayburn

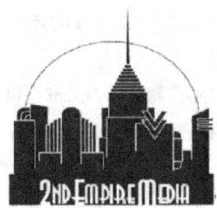

Important Notice!

The information and/or products outlined in this book is designed to be used in conjunction with, not instead of, your doctor's program. If you have an illness, then seek a doctor's care.

Do not use this information as a sole therapy against any disease or medical condition.

The information contained in this book is not recommended to diagnose, treat, cure or prevent any disease.

To purchase the original 30 day program material please visit:

The30DayBurn.Com

About The Author

Danial Barron Howe is the author of over 350 books ranging from business to health and wellness. He is the founder of six multinational businesses including 2ndEmpireMedia, the publisher of this book.

Danial holds several degrees including a Masters in mechanical engineering and design as well as degrees in psychology and biomechanics. He is a lifelong tinkerer with a passion for improving efficiencies of systems such as those found here in this book.

INDEX

CHAPTER 1

Each one of us walking the face of the earth is made up of an abundance of fat cells throughout their bodies. In fact if you're a normal healthy adult with a typical body composition, you have approximately 30 billion of them. This is an astounding number when you think about it. Have you ever wondered why you need so many? Have you ever wondered what all those fat cells are for?

Fat Cells Are Genetically Programmed

The reason is, those fat cells are built into our genetic makeup and they enable us to use stored energy when food supplies run low. This storage mechanism works exactly the same today as it did over 10,000 years ago. However, these days we find ourselves with an abundance of food in modern society, and we no longer need this built in mechanism to store so much fat in order to survive.

When you consume an excess of calories, your body goes right into storage mode for those anticipated "hard times," ahead, but those times never come. So your body simply hangs on to those extra calories in the form of fat. Conversely, when you eat fewer calories than your body demands, your cells will release this stored fat to maintain energy. It all looks good on paper; but, as you will soon see, not all fat is the same.

The Location of Fat Deposits in Your Body

The location of fat deposits in our bodies will vary depending on each person's genetic makeup, nutritional intake and level of activity. Men generally tend to store their fat in their midsection and chest. Women classily tend to store it much lower - around their hips, butt, thighs, and on the back of their arms.

A full explanation of hormones as they relate to fat storage is beyond the scope of this small book, but for now I'll suffice it to say that certain hormonal processes play a large part in determining body fat distribution.

The Prime Factor in Failing to Lose Fat

Many people who attempt to lose fat fail to take into account one major factor, it's a stumbling block to every dieter's long-term success. A vast majority of beginning dieters attack fat loss and fitness with great enthusiasm and determination in the beginning, they get initial positive results and feel great. Even so, they just can't ever seem to get rid of *all* the unwanted fat. They'll lose successfully for a time, but then ultimately find themselves at a *sticking point* just before all of the fat is completely gone.

This is sticking point is known as a *plateau*, and this predictable phenomenon causes many people who were enjoying terrific success to lose their critical focus and enthusiasm and slide back into their old habits. When those old ways take over again the fat comes back with a vengeance. This again, is due to genetic programming of our fat cells. With each new time you attempt to lose body fat, it seems to take longer and demand more and more effort.

Finding the Solution to Stubborn Fat

So where can you find a real solution? The answer to that is simple: you must understand how your bodies' fat cells work and how to break through the *plateau phenomenon* to lose that last bit of unwanted fat—what

I refer to as *"stubborn fat."*

I have worked with thousands of clients over the years and I can say that the majority of them display a good amount of this stubborn fat. Science tells us this type of fat is actually *hardwired* into our basic survival system so as to be incredibly difficult to remove. It appears to stick with us no matter what we do, hence the term "stubborn fat".

Most popular diets and weight loss programs work to one degree or another in the beginning, but they *never really* confront this critical part of the fat loss cycle — removing the last bit of stubborn fat!

Hormones and Their Role in Stubborn Fat

Difficult to remove fat deposits occur when your hormonal pathways brake down. Your also age plays a role in this process as well. It's no secret that fat increases with most people as you get older, largely due to lower metabolism and reduced activity levels. This you have limited control over, but there are still things that lead to stubborn fat accumulation that remain under your control. The choice to reject Yo-yo dieting schemes is one of them.

Losing weight with *crash diets* and then regaining it all again —referred to as "rebounding"—ultimately only increases the tenacity of stubborn fat in the long run. A decrease in exercise and activity level also compounds the stubborn fat problem for most as well. This is why people who go on crash-diets that temporarily radically restrict calorie intake and refuse to adopt the habit of exercise on a regular basis often have the worst stubborn fat problems of all.

Our ancient ancestors never had to deal with this problem. They were constantly on the move and engaged in physical labor as a necessary means of simply surviving, whereas these days technological advances and modern convince has allowed many of us to remain far more sedentary, our food comes *to us* – we no longer need to go get it if we choose!

Stubborn fat metabolizes very slowly and it resists the hormonal processes that takes place when the fat burning process begins. When burning fat, the *adrenal hormones* (commonly known as noradrenaline and adrenaline) attach themselves to fat receptors they basically "crack them open" so the fat inside can be used in the energy pathways.

There are two types of receptors found in your fat cells: the first is alpha, the other beta. Beta receptors display higher activity and respond in conjunction with adrenal hormones. To lose fat, the adrenal hormones fire up and the body begins to convert fat to energy. In situations involving stubborn fat this does not occur, so zero fat is lost.

According to Ori Hofmekler, author of *The Warrior Diet*, stubborn fat possesses a lower ratio of beta to alpha receptors. Therefore, adrenaline - which is your body's "fat dissolver", is unable to make its way into the fat cell to open the door. Hofmekler goes on to point out that "to make these matters worse, stubborn fat has more estrogen receptors, which cause *even more* stubborn fat."

If all this news doesn't sound bad enough, it gets worse, if you indulge in the typical western diet and lead a sedentary lifestyle, you are setting yourself up for *insulin sensitivity*. If this happens your fat tissue becomes even more incredibly resistant to your attempts to lose it, making it appear as if you will be stuck in your "fat suit" forever.

Why Dieting Alone Doesn't Work

Diets generally fail because most only look at the caloric reduction side of the equation. You must also understand the other variables in the equation, namely exercise and proper lifestyle.

Ridding yourself of stubborn fat (for a lifetime) is not nearly as simple as just slashing calories and dieting. Stubborn fat results from a complex interplay of hormonal and biological processes—each of which are positively or negatively affected by how you eat, how you move, and the type of life you live.

The Critical Question

Now that you have a basic understanding of why you have stubborn fat, the question is: *How do you make personal changes that will bring positive results?*

That answer is coming up in Part 2. Read on...

CHAPTER 2

The Curious Differences In Men And Women

The differences are obvious when it comes to the physical make-up of men versus women.

Most Men are 10–15% larger than women on average and weigh about 20% more. Most are 30% stronger too (Especially when we're talking about upper body strength).

Testosterone is the major player of the hormones active in men's bodies. Testosterone drives muscle enlargement and stimulates bone growth, it also has been shown to raise levels of red blood cells in a man's blood stream as well. And while we're at it, let's not forget it plays a key role in the male libido.

Men also produce more human growth hormone (HGH for short) too.

What you may be unaware of, however, is that all of these factors combine to make oxygen far more available to a man's cells than a woman's cells. The result of this is that a man may be only producing effort at 50% of his total capacity during physical activity, but a woman would need to work as high as 70% of her possible capacity just to keep up. It's simply not as easy for her cells to absorb oxygen.

At first this may seem unfair until you consider the reason. Women have a smaller percentage of *lean tissue* and a much higher percentage of body fat to start with. Even though this can be a hindrance in events such as a short sprint, having a higher percentage of body fat means that these same women can power their activities longer from their body's reserves without stopping to eat, drink or to refuel - translating into superior overall endurance.

Repeated studies comparing the sexes in running, swimming, and even skating have shown that the ratio in time vs distance decreased between men and women the longer the event progressed.

Continued research has demonstrated some rather curious differences between men and women in virtually every area. Reviewing the research, you would discover all kinds of random facts such as; women are twice as likely to wear a seatbelt when riding or diving a car than men, to how often they are they tend to be the sexual initiators in a monogamous relationships (that's 65% of the time for those that must know).

As intriguing as these facts may be, let's continue to focus on the differences between men and women that affect women's physical fitness. These differences mainly stem from the functioning of a woman's hormones and function of her fat cells. Together these two factors dictate everything from the way her metabolism functions to how likely she is to experience issues with stubborn fat as well as other health-related diseases, most notably - osteoporosis.

Two Types of Enzymes That Dictate Fat Storage

At first glance the makeup of male and female fat cells is basically the same, but they differ a great deal when it comes to size and function. Women's fat cells are up to five times bigger than their male counterpart! In addition to this, women's cells are not only capable of holding on to more fat, they are genetically programmed to do so*. It all comes down to enzymes:

- **Lipogenic**—are fat-storing enzymes
- **Lipolytic**—are fat-releasing enzymes

sorry for the bad news ladies!

Even though we can find these enzymes present in both men and women, women's bodies contain as much as *two times* the number of lipogenic (fat-storing) enzymes, but only half the number of lipolytic (fat releasing) enzymes. The genetic role of women as the childbearing gender of the species necessitates that this be so. Nature wanted to ensure that women carried enough fat cells to nurture their growing babies and to breast-feed them after they were born. A developing baby requires the mother to burn at least 300 extra calories a day, and later on -breast-feeding can demand as much as 500 extra calories.

In addition to supplying the ongoing caloric needs of a growing baby, our foremothers also developed the ability to store additional body fat in case of drought or famine. As you well know, this extra fat is stored in the hips, thighs, and buttocks. As evolution and history played out, the females who survived famines and droughts got to pass down their genes. Skinny thighs might look good on a cover model but, in the past they were a serious liability, serving only to increase the risk of death when food supplies became scarce.

In a healthy person these enzymes tend to be balanced. An abundance of either type develops an unbalanced system and triggers insulin resistance, a well known contributor to stubborn fat.

Other Contributors to Stubborn Fat

Other contributors to stubborn fat are estrogenic compounds known as xenoestrogens. These chemicals are the byproduct of the fertilizers,soy isoflavones, certain herbs, plastics, and even petroleum products that make up a part of every day in our modern lives. These compounds are found in our food and water supply and they falsely replicate estrogenic functions and aid in binding to estrogenic fat receptors. This produces *"induced aromatase influence."*

Aromatase is an enzyme that promotes androgen (a male hormone) conversion into estrogenic compounds. When this occurs, it magnifies the production of estrogen, which is the main culprit in stubborn fat gain in both men and women. Look around at many of the children today and you can see that they have taken on some very feminized features such as breast fat and take note of the lack of *"manly men"* that seem to be missing from our culture (as compared to only a mere 50 years ago!)

Identifying Estrogenic Compounds

To reap the benefits of a program that reduces stubborn fat, its important to recognize that estrogenic compounds are all around us (and in us). To combat this problem, you should take a hard look at the foods you are consuming and the liquids you are drinking, inside you'll discover many culprits that are causing your stubborn fat problem.

You'll begin gaining stubborn fat the minute you develop bad eating and lifestyle habits. Once this happens you will trigger insulin resistance, a toxic type of overburden on the liver, and elevated estrogen will follow. This chain reaction contributes to fat that will not go away easily. To open these cells up, you need to start by looking further down the food chain.

- Minimize or eliminate all refined foods
- Eat plenty of fruits and vegetables (preferably organic)
- …and exercise.

It's really that simple*…

*Note; I said SIMPLE – I didn't say EASY…Life has no meaning for me without my beloved Oreos, but for the greater good sometimes ya gotta do what ya gotta do! I did it – you can do it too.

In Part 3, you will learn in more detail how to get this stubborn fat out of your life once and for all.

CHAPTER 3

Your Hormones Can Contribute to Stubborn Fat

As you now know from chapter 1 & 2, your hormones can be a real liability when it comes to getting rid of that stubborn body fat.

The estrogen hormone has quite a unique relationship with the fat cell in that it can release signals that actually tell your body to synthesize *more estrogen* or instruct it to regulate the reproductive cycle.

It's been known for a long time that estrogen affects fat cells too. A surplus of estrogen in the body from toxic food sources such as those mentioned earlier can cause fat cells to expand (yikes!) and in turn, become the dreaded stubborn fat you seek to rid yourself of.

A similar situation occurs during pregnancy and in breast-feeding mothers, as estrogen causes the fat cells in the body to swell up so as to absorb and store more fuel for future use.

Estrogen sends out the instruction to stock up on extra fat, so the fat cells unquestioningly follow this order. This is why so many women are shown to gain weight when undertaking the use of birth control pills or when beginning menopause- a time when progesterone levels fall and estrogen becomes the dominant hormone.

Estrogenic Foods Also Affect Men

We've known for years that women naturally have a more difficult time losing fat than men and you have just learned the reasons why. However, men are quickly losing the battle more often in this day and age as well because of the increased exposure to *estrogenic foods* they are consuming in the form of refined foods along with various *environmental pollutions* covered earlier in this book.

Ironically, the biggest reason women have a more difficult time with fat loss than men is because, at any given time, they are more likely to be taking part in the latest fad diet or self-imposed restricted diet intake in order to attain the *model body* that's been established in the west as the new standard of beauty in our culture.

How Dieting Affects Fat Storage

Understand this, severe and prolonged dieting shuts down the metabolism, sending the body into starvation mode*. The fat cells begin locking down output and sending out even more fat-storing enzymes as a frontline defense. Because the fat cells are afraid of being starved to death and depleted of their vital stores, they will use every trick in the book to hold on to the fat they have, causing your body to start burning lean muscle mass all the while reducing your energy levels to practically nothing – all in an effort to preserve the reserves it has for as long as possible.

** One of the greatest diets to take this into account (and it actually really works) is **The30DayBurn**. You'll learn how to lose any amount of weight you want without triggering the fat cell lockdown effect.*

Lean muscle mass is the metabolically active part of the body it is located in the skeletal muscles and the organ systems. What this means is that when your diet is over and your body is no longer in starvation mode, your metabolism will still not function as it did before the diet. This is because you have given up some of your muscle mass, which was the key to driving your metabolism.

In addition, ***the effects of restrictive dieting on your fat-storing and -releasing enzymes can be permanent***. Even though most levels will return closer to a normal level after a diet, the fat releasing enzymes will always be at a slightly lower level than before the diet, and the fat-storing enzymes will almost always be at a slightly higher level. Even worse: ***the effects are cumulative***. What this means is that after each successive round of dieting, it will become harder and harder for you to lose fat and control your weight over the long term.

Don't Panic -There's a Solution!

It sounds pretty hopeless doesn't it? Don't panic just yet! All this bad news doesn't mean that you're stuck with unwanted fat and excess weight for the rest of your life. It only means that you don't have to diet anymore.

Even if you tortured yourself in the past with deprivation diets that left you hungry, anxious, and feeling unhappy, what we now know about enzymes, hormones, and fat cells can actually turn out to be good news. So, *Yes! You can lose your unwanted fat through good old fashioned nutrition, calorie-burning, and metabolism-stimulating exercise and anti-estrogenic foods, and you're about to learn how.*

What I'm suggesting here is not a *magic bullet* type of solution, so if you've been a long-term chronic dieter, it might take a little longer for you than others to make that perfect weight. But by putting an end to chasing quick-results, crash-dieting and choosing to take the weight off gradually, you will not only avoid the feelings of deprivation that undermine most dieters, but all that weight you lose will be up to *three times more likely to stay off* in the long run.

To improve your results in losing your stubborn fat and to reduce the estrogenic effects on your body, there are a few steps you *must* take to ensure your success. Your success depends on understanding how to detox your liver, eat foods that aid in reducing estrogen, and exercising on a consistent basis.

The Stubborn Fat Reduction Plan

On my stubborn fat reduction plan, you are going to consume as many *anti-estrogenic* foods as possible while eliminating as many estrogenic foods as you can.

In addition to stimulating greater fat loss, this type of eating will also help to detoxify your liver.
Without cleaning out the liver and reducing its chemical build up, your liver becomes overburdened, progress stops and your fat loss will hit the wall.

There are a few stages in stubborn fat removal.
Ready? Here we go…

Overview of the Plan

First and foremost you must eat *unprocessed foods* such as fruits, vegetables, legumes, nuts and seeds, and even the occasional wild salmon. This will start the detoxification process for the liver as you eliminate all processed foods, grains, farm-fed livestock, and chemically altered foods that have built up over time. You should try to eat as much organically produced food as possible. If you have a farmers market close by, grab a shopping bag or two and go stock up!

The backbone of your *anti-stubborn fat plan* is to consume large amounts of *cruciferous vegetables* such as broccoli, cauliflower, cabbage, and brussel sprouts. These veggies have been found to be very *anti-estrogenic*. Be sure to include citrus fruits as well such as grapefruit, oranges, and pineapple, because they have enzymes in cofactors that aid your body against radical damage and help your liver detoxify.

If possible, supplement your diet with omega-3 fatty acids from salmon and flaxseed. You may also take an omega-3 fatty acid supplement such as Carlson's oil if you wish.

Eating raw nuts and seeds, avocados, and using olive oil also improves your body's function. In addition, eating green leafy vegetables, whole oats and barley, legumes (*soy is a big no-no!*), and spices such as turmeric (a proven cancer fighter), milk thistle (a great liver detoxifier), dandelion root (an all-natural diuretic), and ginger increases the loss of stubborn fat by lowering estrogen levels in your body.

There are several estrogen inhibitors that will help you rapidly decrease body fat. According to Ori Hofmekler, consuming these foods can not only greatly improve your ability to remove stubborn fat but they can decrease estrogenic effects as well.

Hofmekler says there are additional estrogenic inhibitors such as chrysin (also known as passion flower), quercetin (mainly onions, garlic), apigene (chamomile), all of these cofactors can work together to detoxify your liver and drive away unwanted fat.

To simplify and organize this information, I've broke the process down into three stages:

Stage 1—Start by Eating Anti-estrogenic Foods and Estrogen inhibitors

- Omega-3 oils
- Wild catch salmon
- Cruciferous vegetables
- Passion flower
- Organic dairy
- Citrus fruits
- Chamomile flower

Stage 2—Additional Foods That Will Promote Anti-estrogenic Hormones

- Raw nuts and seeds
- Rice germ oil
- Wheat germ oil
- Olives and olive oil
- Avocados

Stage 3—Foods That Serve as Cofactors and Promote Liver Detoxification

- Fruits (citrus, berries, apples, pineapple)
- Spices (turmeric, oregano, thyme, rosemary, and sage)
- Herbs (dandelion root, ginger, alma berries, milk thistle)
- Green vegetables
- Whole oats and barley
- Legumes (Remember: *No Soy!*)

The Three-week Plan

The following outline is a easy to follow plan that will produce excellent initial results in just a few weeks. After the initial three-week phase, you may then began to rotate the stages as you wish to get continued and even better results.

You may also alternate the stages by the day after the first three weeks.

Stage 1, One Week

Detox your liver

Stage 2, One Week

The High fat for fuel changeover

Stage 3, One Week

Food reintroduction

The Importance of Exercise

In addition to eating the proper anti-estrogenic foods to remove stubborn fat, it goes without saying that you can't cut corners if you are serious about achieving positive results. A crucial part of any diet program is exercise. Diet alone is never enough. Regular exercise is not only beneficial for fat loss, but also for your overall health. Exercise lowers body fat, blood sugar, blood pressure, and cholesterol. You need to set some goals and plan to exercise on a continual basis. Nothing huge, 3 times a week for 30 minutes if that's all you can do but by all means – *DO IT!*

If you attempt to lose weight without exercise, you should expect only temporary success and expect to succumb to the rebound effect. I'm warning you now because if you do not heed my advice, sooner or later you will eventually gain back what you lost - *and more!* And it only gets harder to remove the next time around.

Increasing Your Activity Level

Instead of relying on a *diet-only* approach, try emphasizing a diet and exercise combination and focus on progressively upping your daily activity level overall.

Here are a few quick and practical suggestions:
- Walk to the store instead of driving
- Go for a bike ride
- Walk upstairs in office buildings rather than using the elevator
- Mow your lawn with a push mower
- Vacuum your carpets every other day
- Tidy up your backyard, basement, or garage
- Park your car at the far end of the parking lot instead of looking for a front row space.
- Take short walks during daily lunch breaks or after you get home.
- Iron your clothes; wash your windows
- …and play with your kids.

These activities are usually not considered as exercise or workouts, but activities like these add up at the end of the day, and they can really work wonders as the effects accumulate over time.

Incorporating a Traditional Exercise Program

Naturally, of course, you should incorporate a structured and formal exercise program of some sort to achieve the best results. While it's true that push mowing your lawn can have positive health benefits and does burn quite a few calories, focused exercise is still a must for really making inroads into reducing the most stubborn fat. .

A great type of routine for your fat loss goals is a *circuit training* program. This robust style of training not only raises your metabolism, improves your cardio ability, and improves overall strength but it is also very time efficient.

Put together a routine of your own that makes use of all the large body parts such as upper legs, chest, back, and shoulders and put them into groups to perform. Be sure to do all of the exercises nonstop. You can also mix your cardio training into your circuit workouts or weight lifting to increase the fat burning effect even more.

A Simple Circuit Program

Here are a few examples of effective and time-efficient circuit "modules" that can easily be performed anywhere with nothing but dumbbells or a Swiss ball.

A1 – Lunges

A2 – Dumbbell 3 Matrix (side laterals, bent laterals, front laterals)

A3 – Dumbbell Flys on a Swiss Ball

A4 – Swiss ball Squats (ball up against the wall)

A5 – Dumbbell Cleans

A6 – Dumbbell Row

Do each exercise in perfect form and repeat for 6–8 reps each then then get on your cardio equipment and go hard for about1–2 minutes.

Rest for about 90 seconds then repeat the next circuit 2–3 more times, as your schedule and fitness level dictate.

The *Real Secret* to Stubborn Fat Loss

There is no doubt you can easily take one or two ideas from this book, put them to work and immediately begin to see improvements in fat reduction. However, the real secret, if there is one, is putting all the pieces together into a comprehensive, healthy lifestyle overall.

The lifestyle suggestions below may seem pretty basic and general, but when combined with what you've just learned in this book, they will have a profound impact on your outcome.

- Don't diet—Eat reasonably but do not starve or deprive yourself; avoid yo-yo dieting.
- Avoid empty calories and processed refined foods like sodas and sweets.
- Eat many smaller meals—Eat light at every meal to keep your blood sugar steady and your metabolism stoked.

- Eat healthy fat—Eat omega-3 fatty acids such as those found in salmon to promote proper hormone function and balance.
- Eat a *lot* of vegetables, focusing on the cruciferous variety.
- Drink lots of water—What can I say other than, "without it, you will die!" Drink half an ounce for every pound you weigh.
- Get both sufficient quality and quantity of sleep.
- Keep your stress to minimum.
- Avoid excessive and chronic use of stimulants such as caffeine and nicotine.
- Exercise—Just a little increase in daily activities will go a long way toward improving your health; add circuits and intervals to knock off the most stubborn fat.
- Have a little fun—Find an exercise program you enjoy and stick to it.

Until we meet again;
Live Blessed!
Danial Barron Howe

BONUS #1 : A Look Inside The30DayBurn

The following is a small sample from
The30DayBurn Weight loss Program
By Danial Barron Howe.

How To Kill A Diet In 3 Easy Steps

The first few days of the program are the hardest for most folks. To get through this initial period it is essential that you use every mental and physical trick in the bag to keep your focus on your goal and achieve your goals. Within a few days though something magical happens – *it gets easier. Things began to normalize and a familiar routine sets in. this is when you know "you've got it".*

Here's a few things that helped me quite a bit get through the hard times. Take these observations seriously because if you do you'll notice things go a lot more smoothly for you.

Diet Killer #1: Underestimating the urge to chew

This is a powerful drive that seems to be hardwired right into our DNA. After all, it's a survival instinct. It's remarkable how powerful this urge really is. If you were to go a couple of days on a straight liquid diet, you would literally begin to get an overwhelming feeling of *depression* (Which in turn would kick in your need to eat to alleviate bad feelings) - the feeling is as if some intangible thing is missing from your life, *that's because it is!*

Because it would be unrealistic for the first time in your life to think that you could just stop doing it *cold turkey* we need a way to satisfy this urge without undermining our plan. The biggest problem with having the urge to chew is we have to have something to *chew on*. This typically leads to munching and munching leads to falling off the program!

Luckily we can solve our need to chew without adding calories by carrying sugar free gum. When you begin to get the "munchies" 9 times out of 10 it's not *true hunger* it's just your body wanting to satisfy its need to chew. The solution? Pop a stick or two of gum in your mouth and watch how quickly the thought of snacking subsides.

Diet Killer #2: Running familiar meta-patterns

Another reason we eat when were not really hungry is because an activity may go hand-in-hand with something we familiarize the act of eating with such as sitting in front of the TV, or going out to a movie.

Our brains, while remarkable, still operate in a primitive "*if-then*" form of basic **meta programming** installed in us by years of input from advertising, social programming, early parental influence and more.

For example: "*If* I go to a movie-*then* that means I need popcorn!"

Well, of course you don't *need* the popcorn. That's ridiculous. But, through repetition and failing to actively interrupt this pattern, over time you may have programmed yourself to *automatically* to reach for that large tub of buttered popcorn when you're taking in the latest Hollywood blockbuster whether you really want it or not!

These *patterns* play out in many different ways hour upon hour all throughout our daily lives. And it's your job to actively recognize them for what they are. *Patterns are not legitimate hunger signals* they are something *entirely different.*

Your focus throughout the next 30 days will be to recognize these patterns and interrupt them before they get started. To do so requires being able to recognize the *trigger*.

Triggers come in many forms. They can be a sight, a sound, or situation. They may even be a person.

For example:
Those of you of a certain age will remember the good humor ice cream man. At one point in time in America legions of these ice cream vendors slowly drove trucks around the streets of America accompanied by a loudspeaker on top playing the familiar good humor tune*. This tune became a trigger in the minds of a generation of children to the point that much like Pavlov's famous dogs, children began to salivate at the sound of the ice cream trucks siren song and they would come running in droves!

Your success for the next 30 days will be dependent upon your ability to recognize the triggers in your daily life and even to proactively avoid them as much as possible.

*Interestingly enough, the stronger the trigger the more durable and long lasting the effect. I wonder how many adults that grew up with the good humor man would still respond to that music even today!

Diet Killer #3: Inconsistent Intake

One of the *classics of diet failure* is the infamous *feast* and *famine* technique. It goes something like this: A person will over eat and to compensate for it will double down on their dieting and restrict their eating for the next day or two to make up. And it never works because you're pushing of the body's natural "*panic button.*"

Your body has powerful protective measures in place to carry you through the *hard times* of no food. These days we don't have such things as "hard times" as compared with our primitive ancestors. But our bodies still operate exactly the same way as they always have.

No doubt you're aware that when you starve yourself your body goes into *power down* mode during this time it does its best to forcefully preserve what it deems to be the last of its reserves for an unforeseen time. Conversely, any massive uptake of food beyond what it deems to be immediately necessary dumps into its backup storage cells (fat) for later use.

It really is a simple system, but the diet industry has you thinking there some bigger mystery to what is really going on.

It couldn't be simpler. **<u>Here's literally everything you need to know to lose weight:</u>**

- Never go longer than four hours without eating *something.*
- Never take in more calories than you burn off on a day-to-day basis
- Be sure to consistently drink water all throughout the day
- Limit your intake of processed, animal-based or unnatural man made foods (that also includes dairy, cheese and bread and oh yes, diet soda!)

**That's it! That's all you need to know… Seriously. If you follow these four rules
you will lose weight – GUARANTEED.**

I refer to these guidelines as the *4 pillars of success* and we will be taking a more detailed look at each of them in the next chapter….

BONUS # 2 : What You Should Know About Sleep

Want to lose up to an incredible 3 pounds in less than 24 hours? Make a point of getting to bed earlier. Researchers from the University of Pennsylvania found that just a few nights of sleep deprivation can lead to an almost immediate weight gain.

Researchers asked participants in a sleep study to at least 10 hours of sleep a night for two days and then followed it up with five nights of restricted sleep and four more nights of recovery. After the 11 day study the sleep deprived group had gained almost 3 pounds compared to the control group putting in 10 hours a night.

The results of this study really shouldn't surprise anyone. When you think about it the main function of sleep is to shift the body's processes from *performance* to *maintenance*. This cycle is critical to proper function. Would you race a car nonstop for 24 hours without ever making a pit stop?

Sleep and fat loss-the hormone connection
Fat can wreak total havoc on your hormones and impair your ability to lose fat. For instance, hormones such as melatonin, serotonin, and dopamine influence motivation, mood, sleep, and hunger cravings. The correct natural growth hormone balance is essential because it handles growth and repair of your body. A deficiency in your hormonal balance promotes fat gain.

Sleep plays a critical role in regulating each of these hormones. It's time for a "sleep overhaul" if you find yourself regularly Googling: *"How can I get to sleep."*

The following list highlights some of the more common sleep-disrupting habits that can sabotage your slumber.

Sleep Mistake #1: Eating too close to bedtime.
Late-night meals and trips to the fridge prevent your body from slowing down during sleep as well as raising your insulin level. As a result, less cell-boosting melatonin and growth hormone are released into your system while you slumber

The cure:
Cut out all food and drink intake 3 yours or more before bed.

Sleep Mistake #2: Sleeping with too much light exposure or napping too close to your digital alarm clock.
Even just a small amount of light can disrupt the release of *melatonin* and, subsequently, the release of growth hormones. Research has also shown *cortisol* to remain abnormally high when sleeping subjects are exposed to light as well.

You should also be far away from *electromagnetic fields (EMFs)* emitted from electrical devices such as digital alarm clocks in your bedroom. These can disrupt the pineal gland and the production of melatonin and serotonin. (On a side note: research has also linked EMFs to increased risk of cancer so better to play it safe than be sorry for more than one reason.)

The Cure: Keep your sleeping area dark. The darker the better and keep electrical equipment at least 6 feet away, if you must use these items. It's best to turn the light display away from your line of sight.

Sleep Mistake #3: Drinking too much liquid before bed.

This can be an obvious one but we've all made the mistake many times. Drinking before bedtime can increase your need for late-night trips to the toilet. Waking up to pee interrupts your natural sleep rhythm and puts your whole body out of whack. If you turn the light on when you go, you also run the risk of suppressing melatonin production making things even more disruptive.

The Cure: Stop drinking three hours before bedtime and use a red night light in the bathroom, if a night light is needed at all (it really works!)

Sleep Mistake #4: Exercising late at night.

During the T30DB program you will not be required to exercise so this shouldn't be a problem while on this program but generally speaking for the rest of the population this one is a huge *"no-no"* for sleep deprived among us.

There is little doubt exercise can certainly help you sleep better, so long as you do it at the proper time (I suggest mid-morning). A late-night workout, especially cardio, substantially raises core body temperature, preventing the release of melatonin. It can also interfere with your ability to relax and drift off to sleep, since it usually spikes noradrenaline, dopamine, and cortisol, which stimulate brain activity, which is not a recipe for a good night sleep (who among us hasn't had the experience of a sleepless night due to mind that won't calm down and stop buzzing away?)

The Cure: Avoid any form of cardiovascular exercise in the final 3-hour period before bed.

Sleep Mistake #5: Too much TV or computer use before bed.
Many folks enjoy watching their favourite TV shows, catching up on emails, or just surfing the net in the evenings, but too much time in front of either screen close to bedtime has also been shown to interfere with a good night's sleep. These activities increase the stimulating hormones noradrenaline and dopamine, which as you now know hamper your ability to fall asleep.

The Cure: Set aside 30 minutes prior to sleep to "power down" and focus on mind-calming activities such as meditation or reading a book (*Not a lighted screen type e-reader or kindle!*) These habits will surely boost serotonin and improve your sleep.

Sleep Mistake #6: Keeping your bedroom too warm.
I know it feels cozy at bedtime, but a bedroom that's too warm can prevent an essential *natural cool down* that should take place in your body as you sleep.

Without this cooling process, melatonin and growth-hormone release is disrupted, that means you won't be burning fat while you sleep or benefiting from night-time repair your bones, skin, and muscles require.

The Cure: Try to sleep in a cool area, ideally below 70 degrees Fahrenheit.

Sleep Mistake #7: Sleeping in tight-fitting clothes.
It's true, your favorite PJs really can actually help you sleep better, but not if they're too tight. It's been shown that tightly fitting clothing at bedtime--even a bra or underwear-- raises your body temperature and this too has been proven to reduce secretion of melatonin and growth hormone.

The Cure: Sleep in the nude and avoid excessive, heavy blankets. If you prefer to wear something to bed, make sure it's light weight, made from breathable fabric and is above all else loose fitting.

Sleep Mistake #8: Failure to open the blinds or go outside in the morning.
Remember, melatonin is supposed to be lowest first thing in the morning. If you stay in darkness, your body will not pick up the signal that the time has come to get up and go.

High melatonin levels during the day leaves you feeling groggy, fatigued and unable to fully wake up properly.

It may also possibly lower serotonin, this leads to depression, anxiety, and those wicked, diet killing hunger cravings.

The Cure: Crack open the curtains and throw open the shutters! Let the light in as soon as you open your eyes. Send a clear signal to yourself that the day has begun!

Sleep Mistake #9: Not getting the right amount of sleep.
New research recently reported that people who regularly sleep 7½ hours per night live longer. The American Cancer Association found higher incidences of cancer in individuals who consistently slept six hours or less or more than nine hours nightly.

Most sleep experts agree that seven to eight hours a night is optimal. However, some people may require more or less sleep than others. If you wake without an alarm in the morning and feel refreshed when you get up, you're likely getting the right amount of sleep for you.

When your sleep is insufficient, your cortisol and hunger hormones both surge, causing a corresponding increase in insulin. You also experience decreases in leptin, melatonin, growth hormone, testosterone, and serotonin, all of which lead to weight gain.

The Cure: Aim for 7½ to nine hours nightly.

Sleep Mistake #10: Going to bed too late.
Staying awake until the wee hours causes hormonal imbalance because it increases cortisol, decreases leptin, and depletes growth hormone. It can also cause

us to eat more, and it messes with our metabolism. Cortisol naturally begins to increase during the second half of your sleep--a small boost at 2 a.m., another at 4 a.m., and the peak at around 6 a.m. If you're just getting to bed immediately beforehand, you're missing out on your most restful period of sleep.

More than half the respondents to the 2005 National Sleep Survey reported they are morning people with higher energy earlier in the day, while 41 percent considered themselves night owls. Evening people were more likely than morning people to experience symptoms of insomnia and sleep apnea, enjoy less sleep than they felt they needed, and take longer to fall asleep.

The Cure: Hit the sack between 10 and 11 p.m.

Going Deeper Into The Program

You've gotten your first taste of my program and I know *for a fact* that if you followed along you've gotten some pretty positive results. That being said, I'm sure you're anxious to keep those results going!

Now is the time to head on over to my website and grab a FULL COPY of the program. I have so much more to teach you and a few free gifts as well.

The30DayBurn.Com

Once again I'd like to thank you for your purchase and I'd like to ask you to take time to leave a positive review for others to finally find a little light in the diet darkness. Your success with this program means everything to me.

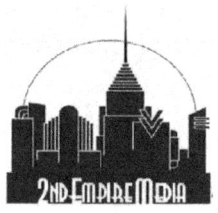

Check out other titles from us

The30DayBurn
The30DayBlast
The30DayCut
The30DayBurn Lifestyle Recipes
and
Many more!

To order visit us at:

2ndEmpireMedia.Com

www.ingramcontent.com/pod-product-compliance
Lightning Source LLC
Chambersburg PA
CBHW070500290526
45790CB00003B/1037